REIKI HEALING MASTERCLASS

The Ultimate Introduction Into the World of Energy Healing, Chakra and Third Eye opening, complete with Guided Meditations

ANNE BRENNAN

TABLE OF CONTENTS

INTRODUCTION

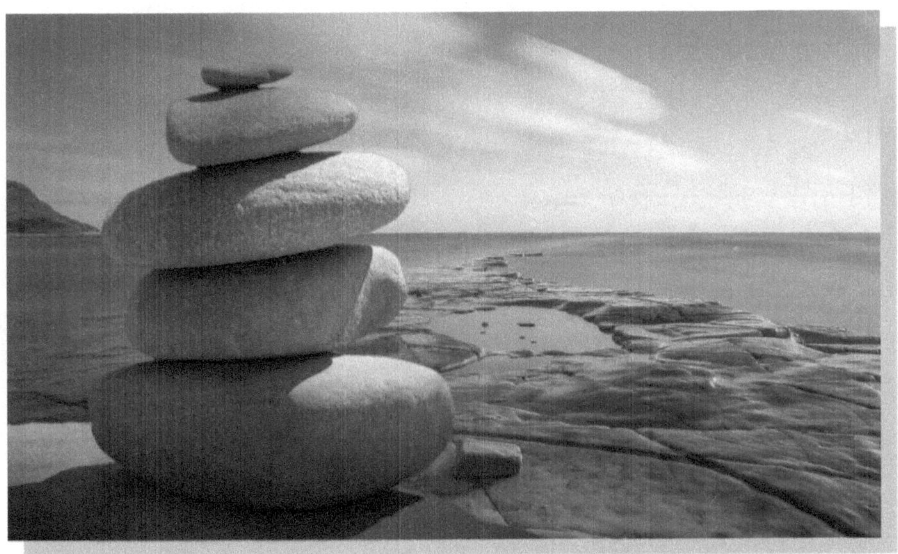

Congratulations on downloading *Reiki Healing Masterclass* and thank you for doing so. The following chapters will discuss the history of *Reiki* and the benefits that you will sustain from practicing *Reiki*. There are also different types of *Reiki* that you will learn about and what you will benefit from each type.

Because *Reiki* is about energy healing, you will also learn things concerning *third eye* and *chakras* and how you can balance them.

Reiki is about guided meditation so you will also learn about a variety of different guided meditation and how you can practice them.

There are plenty of books on this subject on the market. Thanks again for choosing this one! Every effort was made to ensure it is full of as much useful information as possible. Please enjoy!

AS A SPECIAL **"THANK YOU"** FOR YOUR PURCHASE, THIS BOOK ALSO INCLUDES A SPECIAL SET OF GUIDED MEDITATION MUSIC TRACKS **"REIKI ARC"**, DESIGNED TO ENHANCE YOUR MEDITATION EXPERIENCE.
A) GO TO BIT.LY/REIKIARC,
B) CLICK ON **"BUY DIGITAL ALBUM"**,
C) ENTER "**0**" AS PROPOSED PRICE
AND PROCEED TO DOWNLOAD THE TRACKS.

CHAPTER 1: THE HISTORY OF REIKI

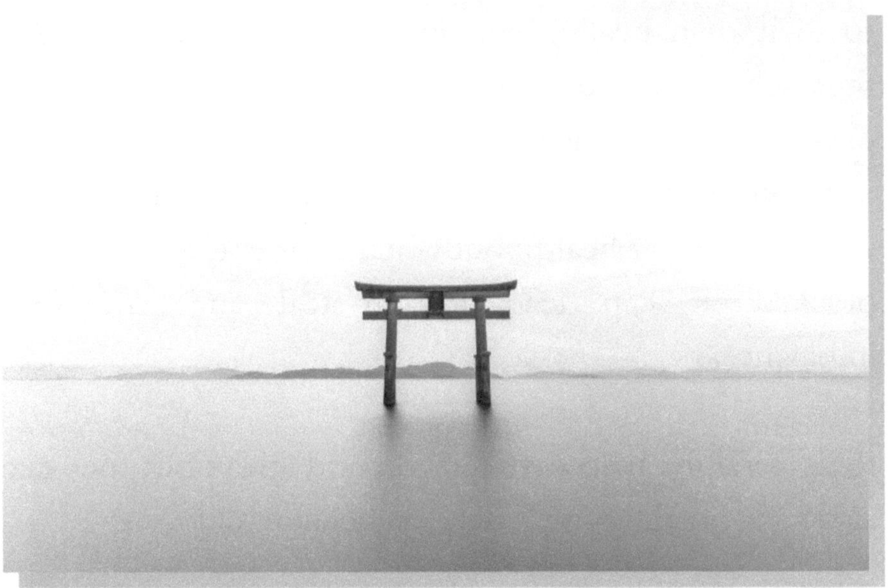

What is Reiki?

Reiki is considered a healing art based in Japan. Reiki comes from the word *rei* meaning "*universal life*" and *ki* which translates to "*energy.*" Reiki is not tied to any specific religion or religious practices nor does it push a specific belief system. Reiki is an effective and subtle form of energy work that uses guided life force energy.

This life energy flows through everything. Reiki practitioners understand that everyone needs to connect to their own healing energy and strengthen it to help themselves and others. Most people believe that a person's energy needs to flow freely. This will be effective whenever a person's mind and body are in a positive state of health; but when their energy is weak or blocked, it can lead to physical and emotional imbalances.

Reiki sessions help ease tension and stress but they can also support the body's need to heal on all levels.

Reiki and Usui

A lot of people think that *Mikao Usui* or *Usui Sensei* was the founder of Reiki and that when he used the word "*Reiki*", he was referring to the healing modality that he discovered and developed. However, whenever you look at the facts surrounding the origin of Reiki, you can see that before Usui developed his particular style of Reiki, there were four other styles being practiced in Japan.

Some time in 1914, a Japanese therapist named Matiji Kawakami developed the Reiki Ryoho which was a healing style that he later published in 1919. During this time, there were other types of Reiki being used. Usui had a mystical experience on Kurama Yama which is where he was gifted with the Reiki energy and where he developed his own style of Reiki which was known as Usui Reiki Ryoho. Usui Sensei picked this name because it indicates that he knows there were other styles being used and this was his own style. But, under the circumstances that developed during World War II and his work with Takata Sensei, the other forms of Reiki were no longer used or remained unknown while Usui Reiki style is practiced around the world.

When we look at what should or shouldn't be considered Reiki, we have to consider that there have been many types of Reiki healing that do not have any lineage starting with Usui Reiki. But, Reiki energy has been around for thousands of years, if not, longer. This energy is something that anyone has the ability to make and use.

However, thanks to the conditions in Japan after World War II, Reiki was brought to the West by Hawayo

Takata; it was Usui Reiki that was practiced as the main form. Because of this, you have to completely understand Usui to understand Reiki.

Chapter 2: The Benefits of Reiki Healing

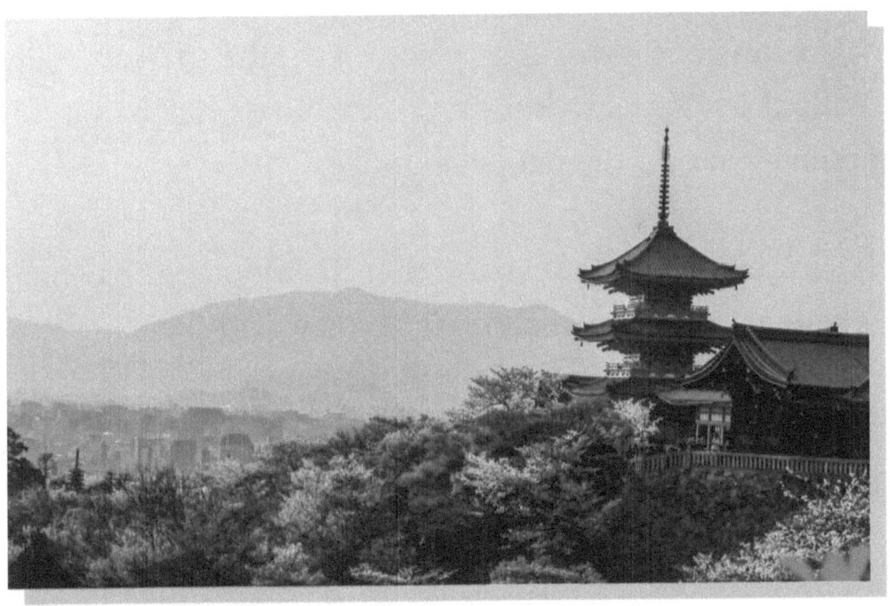

Because Reiki is a healing technique, therapists use it to channel energy to their patients through touch. They are activating the natural healing process that is already inside patients' body in order to help re-balance their emotional and physical well-being.

Treatment like this makes the patients feel as if there is a glowing radiance flowing through them and around them. It is a simple and natural method of healing that is going to complement other techniques that may be used by the patient's doctor or any other therapeutic techniques that they may be applying to their life.

Reiki sessions will take place with the patient fully clothed as the practitioner places his or her hands on various parts of the patient's body.

It's important to understand that Reiki practice balances a patient on every level. Patients may find that they feel refreshed and at peace after they experience a Reiki session. Below I'm listing some of the crucial healing benefits of Reiki:

Reiki promotes of health and well-being through energy healing

-

It can help with pain management because patients are using their energy to help reduce the pain.

-

Patients experience mental clarity because they are being forced to push all the negativity aside to focus on the positive energy.

-

While pushing out all the negativity, patients will experience a release in tension and stress.

-

Patients using Reiki will see that their depression is relieved.

-

Patients using Reiki will also notice that they have a lower anxiety level.

-

It helps patients to experience a state of relaxation through energy healing.

-

Due to the relaxation that the patients will experience, they will also notice that they are able to sleep better.

-

With energetic healing, patients will notice that their digestive system runs smoother than it did before.

-

Without all of the negativity running around inside the patients' head, they are able to have higher self-esteem.

-

Reiki helps to heighten patients' self-awareness because they will understand what is going on in their body.

-

With Reiki, patients can find support for substance abuse and get help recovering from it.

-

It helps promote harmony and balance because it is enhancing the body's natural healing ability.

-

Reiki helps get rid of energy blocks and helps promote the natural balance found between the mind, body, and spirit.

-

Reiki helps clean the body of toxins while supporting the immune system. Because many patients find that they are in a fight-or-flight phase so much, their bodies tend to return to their natural balance. With Reiki, our bodies are reminded to shift into self-healing mode.

-

Patients' self-healing ability will be able to start so that they can return to the natural state. Even if patients do not get to this natural state instantly, they will be pushed in the proper direction. This helps blood pressure and heart rate to improve.

-

Reiki helps with spiritual growth and emotional cleansing because it addresses the entire person instead of just addressing specific symptoms.

CHAPTER 3: TYPES OF REIKI HEALING

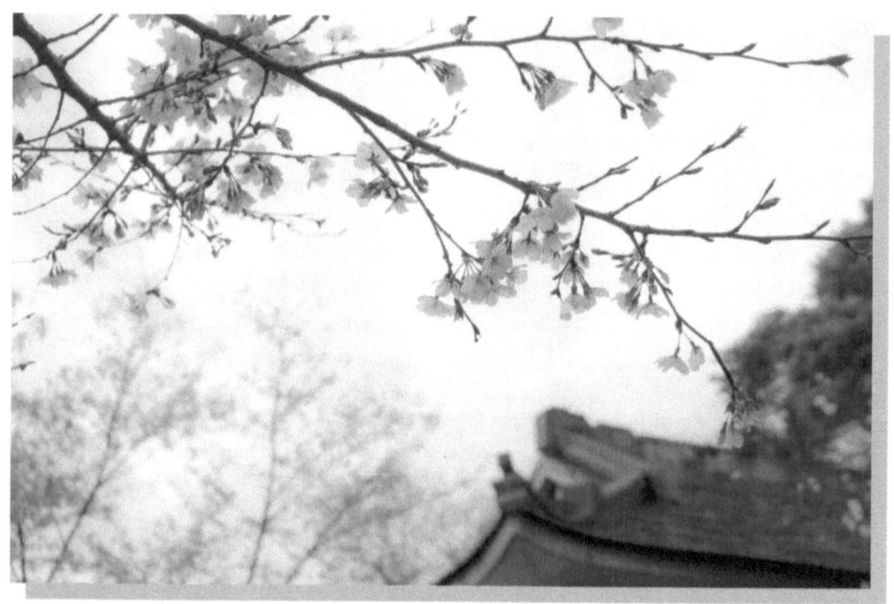

As we discussed previously, there are different types of Reiki that date back years before the Usui Reiki while others are adaptations of Usui Reiki. Each method uses different symbols; however, the principle behind them is the same. In this chapter, you will learn some of the most commonly used Reiki methods.

Usui Reiki

This is considered the first form of Reiki that was brought to the modern world in 1922 by Mikao Usui. It was Hawayo Takata, a Japanese-American born in Hawaii, who brought the Usui Reiki to the West. There have been many changes to the original version of Usui Reiki Ryoho, which is what we know it as now. Usui Reiki differs from how it was taught originally.

Karuna Reiki

Karuna is a Sanskrit word that can be found in the Hinduism, Zen, and Buddhism. This word means compassion. This Reiki healing was created by William Lee Rand, who was the president of The International Center for Reiki Training. This type of Reiki is usually used when trying to relieve the suffering of others. It involves chanting to strengthen the process of healing.

Rainbow Reiki

This type of Reiki was created some time in the 90s by Walter Lübeck, who's a Reiki master in Germany. It is based on the Western teachings of Usui Reiki. With

Rainbow Reiki, new techniques have been created such as chakra work, karma clearing, and inner child work.

Kundalini Reiki

Kundalini Reiki focuses on raising healing energy through the first chakra instead of using the crown chakra. Ole Gabrielsen, a Master of Meditation from Denmark, introduced this method. Kundalini is typically practiced with yoga and can get rid of any blockages that your chakras have. It helps to promote greater peace and strengthen.

Choosing the Right Reiki

While the four types of Reiki we just discussed are not the only ones out there, having such a wide variety to choose from can confuse those that are new to this type of healing. So, how do you figure out which Reiki you should use?

Using Usui Reiki is going to appeal to the traditionalists because it is considered to be the original style. However, some say that there are types that have developed since Usui Reiki have improved on healing. There have even been some students of Mikao Usui who made changes to what their teacher invented to create their own style of Reiki.

Every Reiki will have its own parameter regarding the use of symbols, attunements, and levels. A lot of people are confused on which one to pick.

The first thing everyone agrees on is that every form of Reiki uses *life force energy*. Some people believe that there are greater and lesser forms of life force energy. But, in reality, there are no types of life force energy because it is a free-flowing energy and can be found in all life forms.

One of the easiest ways to visualize life force energy is to visualize water. If you do not have water, you do not have life; and without life force energy, there cannot be life. And just like there are different types of water, the underlying principle is that water provides life to those around it.

Now, remembering that water is water and Reiki is Reiki, you can start to understand that it is not always going to appear that way. For example, you can have a bowl of room-temperature water and in that bowl; you will see different forms take place like the water being frozen or turning into condensation. No matter what form it is in, it is still going to be water.

On the other hand, water takes on many different "attitudes". Water can be soft and gentle or it can be a powerful force like a hurricane or a tsunami.

Much the same as water, Reiki goes on forever and has many forms. It can also be experienced as a gentle storm or a powerful force. Since you can experience Reiki in so many different ways, every type is considered a legitimate way to experience the healing it can provide.

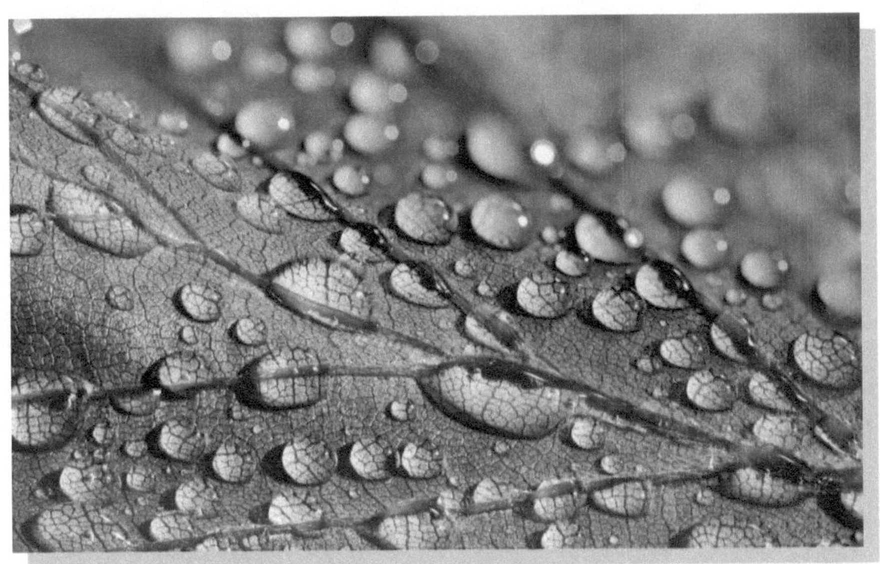

You will know what type of Reiki is for you based on the experience you want to have with the energy and what form you are searching for in your life. Take for instance, Reiki may be *too powerful* for you because you need a *gentler approach* or you could be looking for something *even more powerful.*

In the end, you won't make the wrong choice because one is not better than the other. The best way to find the right Reiki for you is to learn about its different types and then allow your intuition to be your guide.

And remember, you can simply speak to a Reiki practitioner so they can help you find the right one for you!

Chapter 4: Reiki and Your Chakra

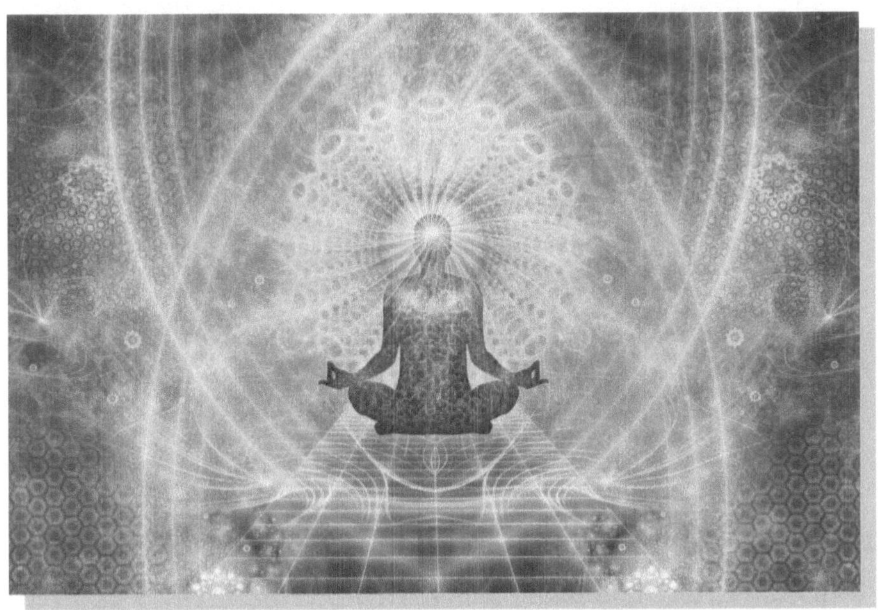

Everywhere around us, there is an energy that is constantly changing. Our bodies soak up this energy like a sponge and it is absorbed through your chakras.

Awareness to the chakras in the human body has been around since before the new age and they play a vital role in yoga.

In Sanskrit, the word chakra literally means "*wheel of light*" and that is how chakras should be looked at as a gift, especially to those that can see them. When someone can see them, they appear as spinning colored light wheels. Each chakra appears as a different color on the rainbow spectrum.

Each chakra is aligned along the spinal column and they form the backbone that connects the body, mind, and spirit. This network includes several smaller energy centers throughout the body and typically corresponds with acupuncture points.

During a Reiki session, the hands will be placed on the major chakras as well as the secondary chakras, which are typically dysfunctional and discolored or even closed off completely because of problems with one's mind, spirit, or body. It is important to keep these gateways open because if there is a disruption in the energy flow, then one may lead to illness.

When Usui developed his version of Reiki, the Japanese culture did not think of the body's energy in terms of chakras. Instead, they were focused more on the hara which is between the pubic bone and the navel. This area will be the center of the body's gravity. There is also a tanden which is in the center of the chest and just above the brow.

But, the understanding of chakras in ancient times added value to Reiki that was practiced around the world. Today, Reiki is practiced everywhere and it takes into account the importance of chakras.

Reiki treatments are supposed to help clear out energy blockages in the chakras while restoring the flow of one's life force energy.

Energy flows in and out of one's aura through the chakras. This aura is a light that envelopes every person. The aura is composed of seven layers, each one dealing with the various aspects of our being. The major chakras create a cone around the core of the spine throughout every layer of our aura.

In one's physical body, each major chakra corresponds with an endocrine gland that helps to control the hormonal balance and a major nerve plexus.

At the base of the spine, there is the root chakra; between the genitals and naval is the sacral chakra; above that is the solar plexus chakra; in the middle of the chest is the heart chakra; in the middle of the neck is the throat chakra; below the brow is the third eye chakra; and at the top of the head is the crown chakra.

There are over a hundred minor chakras in the body as well that play into Reiki.

Balancing Chakras

When your chakras are balanced, you will feel more at peace. You may notice that your chakras are out of balance when you begin to feel ill. Here are some techniques you can use to balance your chakra with Reiki.

Place one hand on the crown chakra and the other on the root chakra.

-

Move each hand closer and further from the body sensing the chakra energy.

If you feel less energy on one of the chakras, then you can use both hands on that chakra using Reiki to bring the chakra back in its original position.

Keep using Reiki until you feel the same with both hands. You should feel a sense of balance so you know that it is fine to move to the next chakra.

The next session will start with your hand over your third eye chakra and your sacral chakra.

You will repeat the same experience until the chakras are balanced.

Continue moving down the chakras until you have finished balancing all the chakras.

You will need to trust your intuition in this process and ensure that you are leaving your patient balanced and calm. When it comes to regular chakra balancing, a person may start to receive insights into issues that are laying inside the deeper layers of the chakras. You have to decide if Reiki is going to be enough to deal with all of these impurities or if another therapy is needed to help balance the patient.

CHAPTER 5: THE THIRD EYE AND REIKI

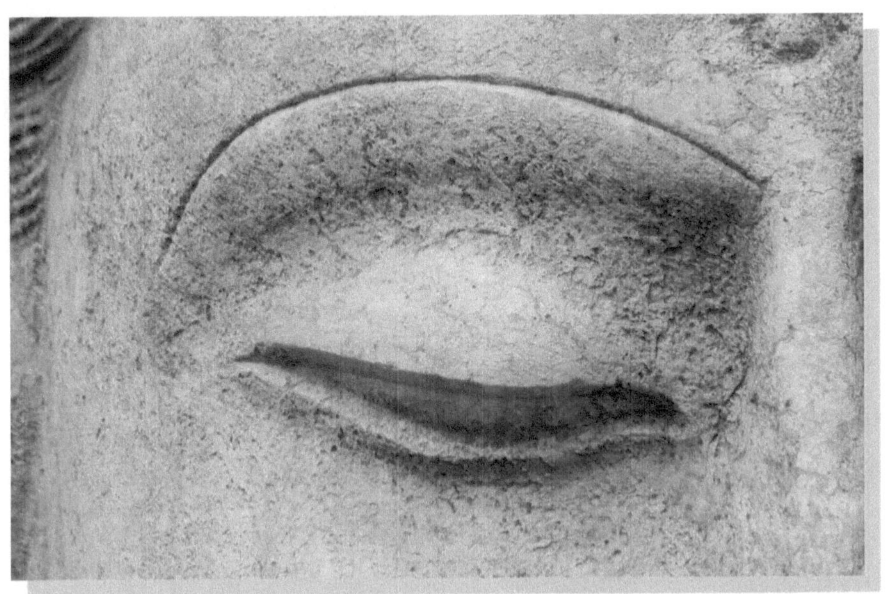

Your third eye chakra is between your eyes and it deals with intelligence and psychic power. The colors associated with the third eye are violet, deep blue, and indigo.

As you perhaps know from biology, *hormones* are responsible for how the body functions. Hormones are tied to many aspects of your body including the physical, emotional, and mental aspects. Modern day Reiki practitioners relate chakras to the *endocrine system.*

Functions of the Third Eye Chakra

For your physical health, the third eye governs the pineal gland along with your eyes, ears, nose, and the skeletal system. It is tied to the senses of sight and hearing as well as one's ability to form their own opinions about the world around them and how they are going to live.

Your third eye secretes a hormone known as *melatonin* which regulates your sleep cycle and growth and also slows down the aging process while maintaining a stable mind. This gland is sensitive to light which makes most people believe that the eyes are stimulated from the pineal gland when melatonin is released. Many scientists think that the electromagnetic field of the earth is also responsible for stimulating this gland.

Your pineal gland governs your eyes and how you see the world around you, as well as any psychic and intuitive abilities you may have.

The third eye chakra plays a vital role in determining how alert you will be, as well as help with how clearly you see things and how optimistic you are while you visualize the outcomes you want. This chakra will create a reality for you that can become real based on your perception. Whenever this chakra is balanced, you will have the ability to visualize better and your memory will become sharper. You should trust yourself that you can be able to rely on your intuitions. You will also be able to help someone without them requesting for your help.

An imbalanced third eye chakra causes problems in understanding reality or creating our own. You may find that you are relying too much on luck and blaming someone when a bad situation happens. Your headache will cause trouble on you which will also lead to having a constant feeling of anxiousness. You may find that you want to dominate or control others. If you experience these things, then your third eye is blocked.

Using Reiki to Unblock Your Third Eye

Reiki practitioners have their own methods of working the third eye chakra. However most often the following basic steps are used to help you clear your third eye chakra with Reiki:

Relax.

Allow the Reiki to flow through you.

Place your hands above your eyes and forehead.

Move your hands in circular motions.

Note, that there are a few that say you should use a clockwise circulation if you are a female and counterclockwise if you are a male. You should allow your intuition to guide you and discover what is best for you.

There are other techniques that you can use as well. *Mantra healing* can be helpful because the repetition and vibration will help to open up the energies in your chakras.

Aromatherapy can clear chakras; if you are using aromatherapy then you should use essential oils such as mint, lavender, and jasmine.

Gemstone healing works with indigo, sapphire, and azurite. You may be able to use other indigo stones as well.

Once again, you should follow your intuition and seek help if you need it. Reiki practitioners can help you clear and balance your third eye.

Chapter 6: Introduction To The Guided Meditations

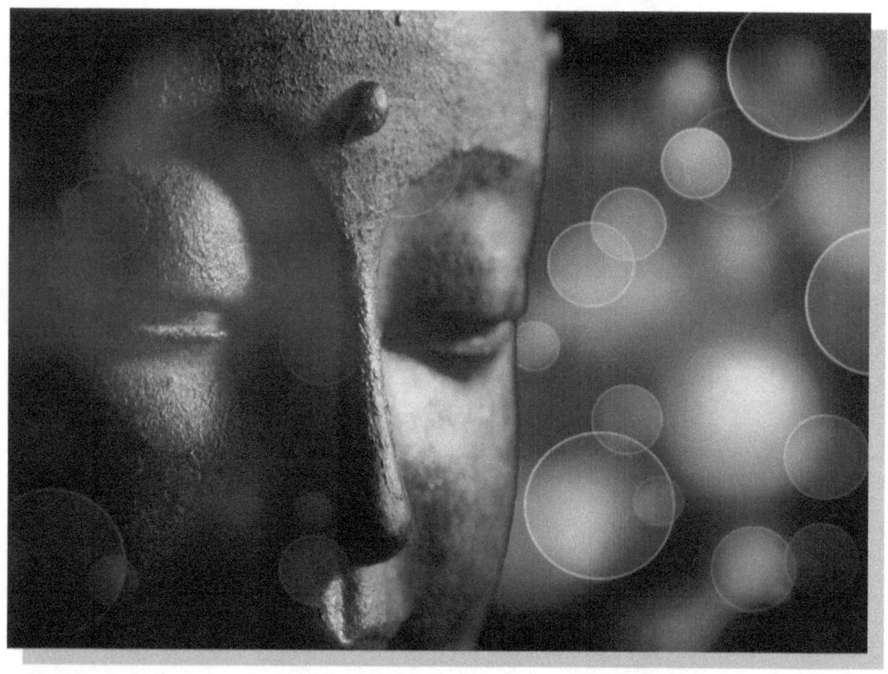

Guided meditation is when you do a meditation usually with an experienced mediator who guides you through your meditation with his voice. He will indicate what you have to do at every moment of your meditation. Most guided meditations have music playing in the background to help you get into the mood of meditation which will be a state of tranquility.

There are some guided meditations that have a specific purpose such as to relieve stress or to generate compassion. Yet, others are there to help you observe your thoughts or take control of them.

Starting meditation can be overwhelming at first, but it can help you to reduce frustration while having someone there to guide you through your first few sessions.

The goal of guided meditations is to make it to where you do not need any external help in the end. Meditation is supposed to be a cold space in your mind where you are alone with your thoughts. Be aware, that in the beginning, meditation is not easy and may seem boring, but that is why you have to take *baby steps* to get to your final goal.

It is recommended that after you get to <u>at least</u> 20 minutes of guided meditation, you should start trying to meditate on your own.

During your guided phase, you should start with 1 minute of meditation and move up. Every day is going to increase until you hit 20 minutes which is when you should begin to feel comfortable enough to meditate on your own.

When you meditate on your own, you need to use a timer to control your meditation. Figure out what type of meditation you want to do and do it without guidance.

Calming meditation: Whenever you feel anxious or agitated, this meditation can help you to calm your body and your mind. Breathe slowly and repeat your mantra to yourself that will help you to bring feelings of well-being and deeper inner peace. Become aware of your breathing and allow your breath to fall freely and rhythmically.

Inner peace meditation: Uplifting meditations are meant to help you fall into a zone of peacefulness. Focus on every breath that you take and release. You should start to feel yourself moving towards a place of inner pace. In the event that you want to cultivate a specific virtue, you should write it down and place it where you will see it every day.

Body scan meditation: With body scan meditation, you will become aware of various parts of your body and become attuned to how each part feels without judgment. You are supposed to cultivate an open and compassionate attitude about your body. You may also focus on wider parts of your body or narrow it down to specific regions. In order to use body scan meditation, you will lie down and direct your attention over each part of your body one at a time.

Loving-kindness meditation: Sit quietly with your eyes closed and your muscles relaxed as you take deep breaths. You should imagine your entire body and feel the perfect love for yourself. Thank yourself for everything that you are and that you know. Repeat several reassuring and positive phrases to yourself. Allow yourself to focus on the positivity flowing around you. If you stray, redirect your attention back to what you are doing.

Breathing meditation: Choose a quiet place to meditate. Sit somewhere where you do not allow yourself to get distracted nor you will become sleepy. Get rid of all distractions and close your eyes. Breathe naturally without trying to control your breathing; you should become aware of the sensations you feel as the air enters your body and leaves. Concentrate on these feelings and nothing else.

Walking meditation: Find somewhere where you feel safe to walk. While you are meditating, you should not become too deep in your meditation that you place yourself in danger. Pay attention to your feet as they hit the ground while you keep the same pace. Allow yourself to think about the goals that you want to accomplish and imagine your stress falling to the ground each time your foot hits the ground.

Focused attention meditation: Focus all of your attention on one thing such as what your goals are. You will need to find a quiet place and visualize what your goal is. The more you focus on your goal, the stronger it will become, which means that the less there will be to distract you from your goals. Just remember that the stronger your visualization is, the more likely you will reach your goal.

Zen meditation: With Zen meditation, you will sit on the floor with your legs crossed, arms in rested position, and hands formed in oval. Focus on your breathing and count how many times you breathe in and how many times you breathe out. You need to also focus on your posture. Most people practice Zen in the lotus position.

Vipassana meditation: Vipassana is practiced like Zen but the difference is that you have to develop a sense of concentration by using a practice known as samatha. Once again, this is usually done by becoming aware of your breathing. Focus on every moment that passes and what you are doing in that moment. You may notice that there are small changes to your breathing that you have never noticed before—like how your abdomen rises and falls or how the air feels as it enters your nose or passes over your lips.

Mantra meditation: This is quite easy to do. You will find a mantra that you want to instill in your mind and you will repeat it as you meditate. The mantra meditation helps you focus on your goals or helps you to bring more positivity into your life.

Transcendental meditation: This meditation type is not usually taught. You will do transcendental meditation twice a day. It is similar to mantra meditation, but you will not be making up your own mantra; you will be assigned one that is based on your age, gender, and where you are in life. This type of meditation has to be learned from someone who is licensed to teach it.

CHAPTER 7: GUIDED REIKI MEDITATIONS

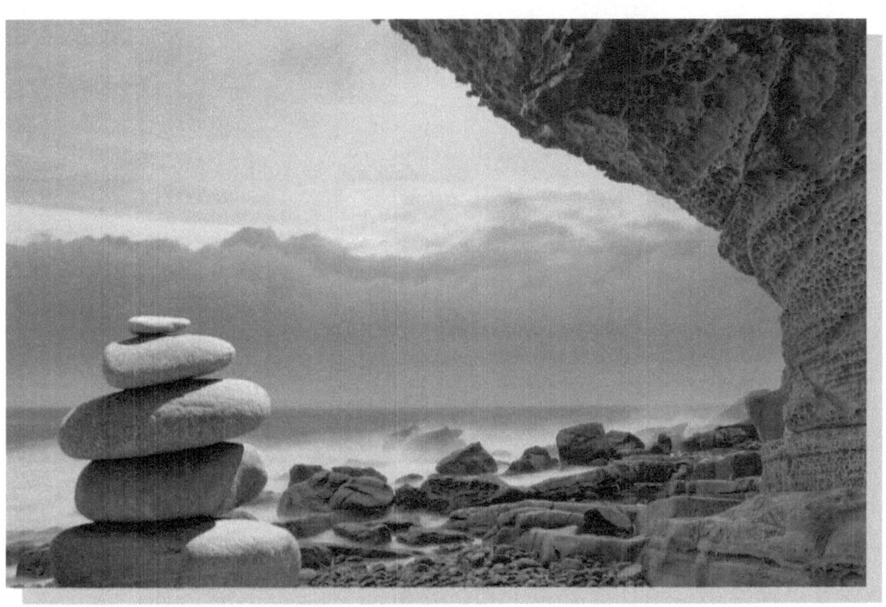

The following guided Reiki meditations are written with you, my dear reader, in mind. They are written so that you can raise your vibrations and nurture your entire being from your mind, body, and spirit. It is my hope that they will be able to help you leverage Reiki to the fullest of your capability.

To use the meditations, set aside a special time for you to mediate. You can go into your special room—it can even be your bathroom or closet. Lock the door, light a few candles, turn off the lights, and get comfortable. Try to clear your mind—and the meditations will help you with the rest of your meditation sessions.

As you listen to the guided meditations, remember to breathe in through your nose and exhale through your mouth. Breathe in your breaths as deeply as possible, and exhale those deep breaths through your mouth as steadily as possible. If you find that you are getting off track, that is okay. Bring your mind back to the meditation as fast as possible.

You will find that the more you meditate, the easier it will become. The meditations in this book focus on helping you enjoy the ability to work hard, developing kindness in your spirit, ridding yourself of anger that is preventing you from becoming the person you need to be, kicking worries out of your mind, and leveraging the warmth that comes with gratitude to help you enjoy your daily path.

Reiki Healing Meditation #1

Get comfortable, and close your eyes.

Today is a wonderful day. It is a beautiful day.

For one moment, listen to the chirp of the birds. Listen to the sound of the cars passing by. Focus on the chirp until you no longer hear it. Focus on the sound of the car as it passes by—and you can no longer hear the rumbling of its motor. Listen to the silence. Feel the stillness in the silence. Embrace the stillness. The stillness is you.

Focus on your breathing. Feel the gentle rise of your chest going up and down softly. Notice the thumping of your heart. Breathe in slowly and deeply. Take in all the great news you are going to receive today. When you inhale, feel all the positive energy spreading throughout every nerve and cell of your body.

Exhale any negative thoughts you may have had today. Exhale all of the negative energy from miscommunication that you may be having. Maybe you are thinking negative thoughts that prevent you from seeing that people *are* just people. Let go of your lofty expectations of others.

Inhale the grace that you want others to give to you. Let that grace affect every part of your being so that you can be gracious. Inhale positive thoughts that will help you speak the exact right thing that you need to say. Inhale the possibilities of gentle words and the power that they have.

Exhale all of the bad things that are not going to happen. They have disappeared. They are no longer there. Inhale all of the positive, amazing, great things that are going to happen to you today.

Know that you are loved—and this is your day. Inhale the goodness of the day. Inhale the possibilities that today could be the very best day of your life. This is the day that will start a domino chain effect of nothing but good things to come for yourself and for others.

Open your eyes. *Brave the day.*

Reiki Healing Meditation #2

You are in your special place. This is a place just for you. You are safe to let go of any doubts or negative thoughts you are having. Let them go somewhere else. You are too full of positivity to make room for any negativity. There is no space within you to entertain something that is not uplifting you.

Close your eyes. Inhale deeply, and feel your breath go as deep into your chest as possible. Let Reiki fill your chest. Think of the abundance you will have today. Think of the extra that you will be able to share with others.

Exhale all of the distractions that are standing in the way of your abundance. They are no longer a factor. As a matter of fact, they are like a whiff of condensation. You can no longer see them. You no longer hear them. You no longer feel them.

Inhale the abundant joy that you will experience. Today is the first day of many abundantly joyful days to come.

Think of everything that makes you happy—children's laughter, the smile of a loved one, the bark of your dog, the purr of your cat, and the smell of a freshly printed book.

Breathe out all of the sad things and bad news that you have heard recently. Maybe someone hurt you. That's okay. Your abundant joy is more than enough to overcome their hurt and yours. Be grateful for Reiki and the ability to overlook negativity.

Breathe in all of the abundant prosperity that you are going to have. Feel Reiki racing to your fingertips, the tips of your toes, your tongue, and your brain. You are what you need to be at this very moment—*revel in it.*

Breathe out any doubts of where you are supposed to be right now. Quiet the noise. Inhale abundance as deeply as possible.

Open your eyes, and have a great day—a day full of everything that your heart desires and a day that is in line with the universe.

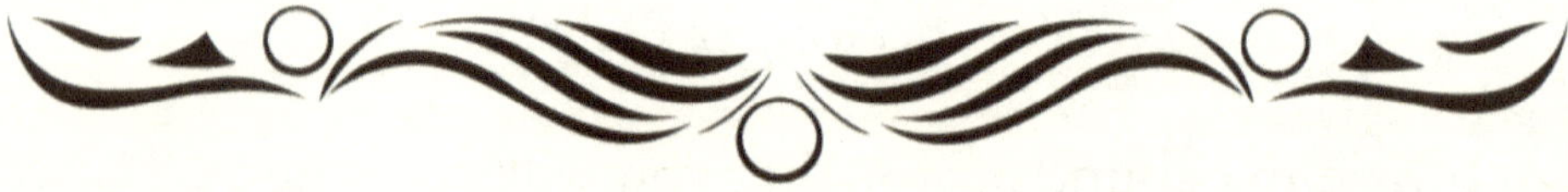

Reiki Healing Meditation #3

There are a lot of thoughts running around your mind
right now
Your mind is racing, but grab that last thought—let it
disappear.

Let all of your thoughts simmer until they have
vanished like a mist in the wind. Take note of the
lightness of your eyelids caressing your eye. Take a
breath as big as you can—and let it all out. Still your
thoughts.

With each breath that you exhale, let worry fly out of
your brain. Replace worry with assurance. The worries
you have are blocking you. With each breath, imagine
your worries weighing less and less—your worries are
becoming lighter and lighter.

When you breathe in, imagine a feeling of completion
and gratitude.

All of your problems have been taken care of.

Take full deep breaths—and rest assured that with every breath, your worries have dissipated into thin air. They vanish. See your strong self while being guided by Reiki, covering all of your steps.

Feel the life force travel through every toe, sliding up your ankle, swimming around in your tummy, jumping up to your chest, down your arms, around your fingertips, back up to your neck, throughout your face, and finally to your head.

Feel it tickle your eyes, encouraging you—empowering you to see the great, worry-free life that you already have. Today, let your worries rest. They will take care of themselves because Reiki is working it out for you.

Let Reiki use you to be gentle and kind and light to others who need you. Do not let things that you cannot change bog you down.

Open your eyes — *make your day a great one.*

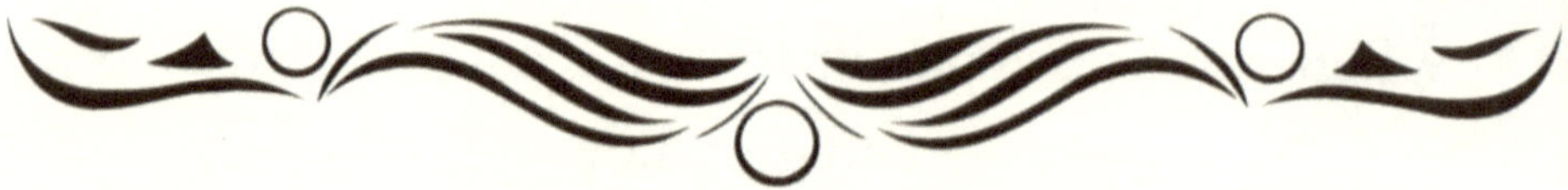

Reiki Healing Meditation #4

When you are comfortable in your special place, slide into stillness. Slide into utter stillness and utmost silence.

Do you feel your breath?

Each breath you breathe tickles your insides, calming your worry. Your worries are no longer insurmountable—they are just gentle obstacles that you can scoot by. Continue to take deep, long breaths—and feel the life force swirling within you. You can breathe out any problems that you think are too big for you to handle until they are now manageable bit by bit.

Today, your goal is to focus on everything that Reiki has provided. With every breath, focus on what you *can* do—not what you cannot do. You *can* be kind and gracious in every relationship that you have. You *can* speak life-affirming words to those around you. You *can* use the power of your tongue to uplift and change your situation.

If you think positive, your body and actions and Reiki follow.

Inhale a gigantic breath. Let your body take in all the positivity that deep breathing brings.

Breathe it out—rid yourself of all your worries.

One more time.

Inhale a humongous breath. Think of the great things that are going to happen today—and breathe out every single one of your negative thoughts.

Now, open your eyes — *face this day with a smile.*

Reiki Healing Meditation #5

Start this meditation by settling and reflecting on an act of kindness you have done recently. Bring your thoughts to that one moment where you gave selflessly.

Imagine how you felt. Feel the Reiki sending positive vibrations throughout your body. Breathe deep and purposefully. Receive the life force equipping you with the spirit of kindness.

Breathe out any mean thought you have—even the smallest of things. Breathe in the spirit of kindness. Breathe in as much kindness as you can. You are kind to spiders, ants, and ladybugs.

You are kind to strangers you pass by in the street and your friends and family members that you love so deeply. You are kind to that one person in the office that no one speaks to. You are kind to the child who is

having a hard time at home. You are kind to someone
at the exact perfect time who needed to have someone
to be kind to them. You are their last hope in humanity.
Embrace the gravity that being kind has.

Breathe out your knee-jerk reactions to rude people.
Breathe and reinforce yourself with the spirit of
kindness to even the meanest person you know. They
are really in need of your kindness. Breathe out how
you want to act to them. Breathe in the spirit of
kindness guiding you to be kind to people—even in
situations where you do not think they deserve your
kindness.

Do you feel your body receive the spirit of kindness?
Breathe steadily and deeply. Do you feel its warmth?
Embrace the coldness and negativity and meanness
exiting your body. Do not let them come back.

You are cloaked in kindness—ready for all the great
doors being kind will open for you—seen and unseen.
Even if you do not gain any material reward from your
kindness, know that Reiki is pleased.

Your path rewards your kindness as you reward others
with your kind words and thoughts.

Breathe in a big gulp of kindness one more—and let go
of anything standing in the way of you being kind.
Open your eyes gently. Blink.

Stand. Start your day, and *be a ray of light to others.*

Reiki Healing Meditation #6

Smoothly shift your body to your most comfortable position. If you are already in your most comfortable position, you can stay there.

Breathe in. Breathe out. Breathe in. Breathe out. Focus on your breaths when you breathe in. Breathe in. Hold it for three seconds. Breathe out. Breathe in from your nose. Gather the breath from the soles of your feet, and bring the breath out through your mouth.

With every deep breath, focus on the hard work that Reiki has allowed you to do. Focus on the benefits of being able to work with your mind or hands to provide for yourself and your family. Be thankful.

Exhale every single excuse that stands in the way of you not being able to do a good job on your work. Get rid

of every mental block that prevents you from showing
gratitude for the work that you are able to do right now.

If you are looking for a different passion or a different
calling—or if you want to continue to excel with what
you are currently doing, inhale the life force. Feel it
guide you to the path that you need to take.

Exhale the particles of negativity, slothfulness,
procrastination, ungratefulness, and laziness.

Inhale the joy of met guidelines and great jobs of
completing your tasks. You are a hard worker—grateful
for Reiki for the opportunity for fruitfulness.

Do not squander the moment to work today for a
better tomorrow.

Breathe out. For one more time, breathe in the joy of a
job well done. Sure, accolades are great—but feel the
joy and pride of knowing that you did the best job that
you could do. Feel grateful that you are being rewarded
for the hard work that you do by Reiki.

Blink three times. Open your eyes, and *be productive and grateful for today.*

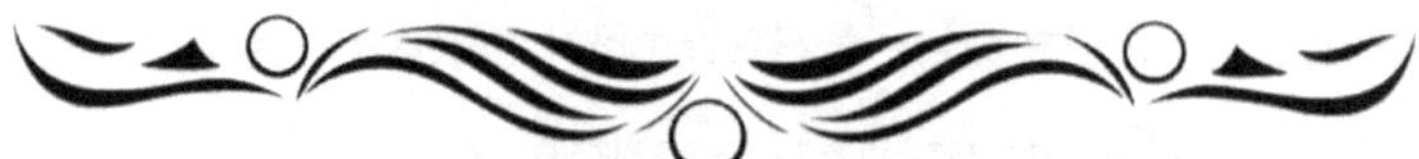

Reiki Healing Meditation #7

Close your eyes, and breathe in deeply through your nose. Exhale the breath through your mouth.

Today, we will focus on the anger and pain that is blocking you from using, enjoying, and surrendering to Reiki. Think of that one thing that has angered you for days, for months, for years. Do you feel how your body reacts to it—the quickened breath, the clenched teeth and hands?

Breathe those feelings out through your mouth. Breathe in, and replace those feelings of anger with feelings of compassion. Breathe out that anger, and breathe in. Replace those feelings of anger with a feeling of understanding. Breathe out the anger, and breathe in deeply. Feel the life force swarming into your body— gently zapping every feeling of anger that you have.

Replace those feelings of anger with feelings of gratitude.

Feel the lightness that overcomes your body. Feel your chest touching your heart when you breathe in. Exhale and feel your chest rise as high to the sky as possible.

You are no longer looking at your situation that angers you through angry eyes. You are now looking at the situation through the eyes of gratefulness for the lessons that you learned. You are looking at it with eyes of forgiveness and forgetfulness.

Breathe out the last of the hurt, anger, and frustration. Breathe out all the negative effects that these horrible feelings have on your body. Watch your health improve instantly.

Inhale the spirit of clarity.

Draw the longest and deepest breath that you can. Exhale the breath slowly, surely, and assuredly. Feel Reiki at work. Feel Reiki giving power to your tongue, your spirit, and mind—preparing you to be great.

Open your eyes, and prepare for a day full of happiness
with no remnants of anger nor any hint of regret — but
with no other than readiness to embrace everything life
has to offer.

Reiki Healing Meditation #8

Collect your scrambled thoughts one by one. Put them in a basket of forgetfulness. Tuck the basket away for the time being. Breathe in and breathe out while you collect your thoughts. Steadily, slow your breaths down until you can only feel your body fill with the Reiki from every deep breath that you take.

Be still. Be calm. For the next 10 seconds, be completely at peace.

Look at the blank canvas of your mind. Think of situations that anger you. Do you see the vivid colors that are splashing on your mental canvas?

Feel your breath steady the white canvas. Exhale any thought and colors that may be coming to paint that canvas. Exhale and push them away until your mental canvas is totally blank.

Inhale slowly. Exhale slowly. Inhale forgiveness. Exhale anger.

You are the master of calm—the painter of forgiveness. On the canvas of your mind, feel the Reiki traveling throughout the canvas and throughout your body with every breath. Each breath steadies your mind's frantic thoughts. Keep the canvas as white as possible.

With every negative thought that wants to overcome your white canvas of calm, dump feelings of forgiveness and understanding and compassion and forgetfulness until the canvas is back to being white again.

Embrace the difficulty of trying to still your thoughts. You know that your mind and Reiki are working. Keep stilling your thoughts. Every hint of anger pops up— run your broad brush of love across it.

Feel Reiki guiding your hands and helping you keep your brush steady—helping you paint with steady fingers and pure heart and kind mind. Feel your body being reinforced by Reiki—empowering you to say all the right things that need to be said and to take all the right actions that need to be taken.

Do you see how white and bright your mental canvas is? Now, splash kindness, understanding, gratitude, and love on the canvas. Keep your mental canvas with you. Know that you can return to this canvas to start over at any time.

Open your eyes, and keep this beautiful mental picture with you.

Reiki Healing Meditation #9

Reiki is so kind. Reiki is so beautiful. Reiki is so loving. Reiki is so compassionate, forgiving, and understanding. Breathe in. Breathe out.

Breathe in kindness. Breathe out meanness. Breathe in beauty. Breathe out ungratefulness. Breathe in love. Breathe out anger and hate. Breathe in compassion. Breathe out misunderstandings and quick-temperedness. Breathe in understanding. Breathe out the need to speak quickly without listening. Take one moment to listen to your heart.

Let your heart's gentle thump match the deepness and fullness of every breath that you are inhaling and experiencing. Breathe out the negativity that is weighing you down and not uplifting to you. You have that right to choose to be happy. You have the right to choose gratefulness every day. You have the right to choose kindness over envy and jealous heartedness.

Your breaths help you mold your being. Your breaths help Reiki fill you with everything that you need to be filled with—what you're aware that you need and even those you don't know that you need.

Be aware of the universe coming together to bring to fruition everything that you need to be successful. Feel it coming together. The deeper you breathe, the more beautiful it will manifest itself for you.

Breathe out any mental blocks from anger and hurt and pain that you are experiencing. Maybe the pain is from a misunderstanding. Maybe the pain is from an unkind word that has stuck with you. Breathe that out. Exhale deeply through your mouth.

Know that you are your breaths. Know that you are capable of doing whatever you want. Know that Reiki has already equipped you what you need. Allow yourself to accept. You are worthy of it. You are grateful for it.

Allow yourself to accept all the wonderful presents that
the universe has for you. You are worthy of it. You are
grateful for it. You are prepared to make the most of
the tools that you are giving. You are open to Reiki's
help.

Breathe in deeply one more time. Breathe out. Let your
eyes slowly open — and embrace the greatness that *is*
you.

Reiki Healing Meditation #10

Gratefulness—you are so full of gratefulness. You have gratefulness pouring throughout your every cell, giving power to your very being.

Control your breaths. With every breath that you breathe in through your nose and breath out through your mouth, control them. Go at a steady, slow pace. Let your breath control your thoughts—do not let your thoughts control your breathing.

Breathe slow. Breathe steady. Inhale. Exhale.

Just like that. Great job. Keep it up.

Go to your favorite place. Feel the goodness, safety, and warmth of that place. Dwell in its goodness. Let the gratefulness of the experience wash over you with every breath that you take.

Now, go with me to a forest—a peaceful forest. This peaceful forest has the tallest trees that reach to the heavens and make you know that Reiki is there to guide you. Breathe in, and feel fortified with the spirit of Reiki. Exhale and go with me to the beach.

Imagine that you are sitting in a chair—exactly where the waves meet the sand. Feel the water tickling your feet. Feel the waves crash between your toes. Breathe in the delight. Inhale all the pleasantness of being at the beach. Feel the warmth of the sun. Let the warmth envelop you. With every breath, feel the warmth of Reiki reaching every limb of your body and strengthening in you—preparing you to handle things seen and unseen.

Go back to your favorite place. Bottle all those warm feelings. Sprinkle your breaths with those warm feelings. Breathe in, and let those sprinkles delight your spirit. Exhale anything that is not in that bottle—doubt, fear, and uncertainty. Be grateful.

Be grateful for the good, the bad, and the ugly. Breathe deeply through your nose. Breathe out, and let the Reiki come in. Fortify yourself with another deep breath.

Flutter your eyes. Open them, and feel gratitude all over your body. Stand and let gratefulness carry you throughout the day.

CONCLUSION

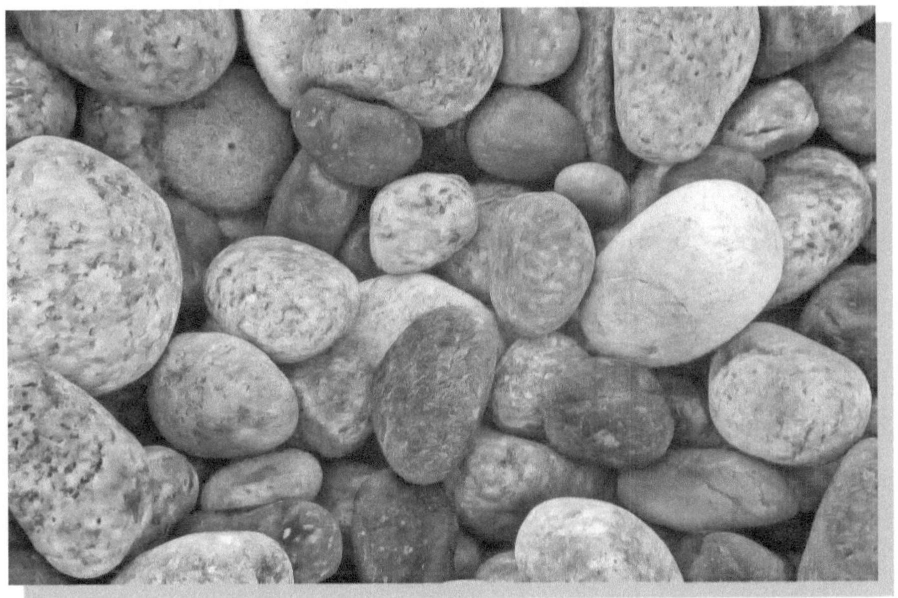

Thank you for making it through to the end of *Reiki Healing Masterclass*. Let's hope it was informative and you learnt enough about Reiki to make it a part of your life.

The next step is to fully embrace Reiki and let it change your life! Reiki can be used to help you heal your mind, body, and soul with life force energy.

The great thing about Reiki is that you can use it with other therapies or anything else that you are using in your life to help make yourself *whole*. Reiki offers so many benefits that you will discover that it can change your life. You will also begin to feel better about yourself and the life that you are living. And, if you do not like the life that you are currently living, then you will be pushed in the direction of changing your life so it becomes what you want it to be.

I also hope that you will continue to develop your Reiki meditation practice. I'd like to encourage you to meditate <u>daily</u>. You can also work on lengthening the time that you meditate. This will surely lead to a major improvement in your life. Remember that the more you practice, the better you will become, and the better you will be able to be a vessel for Reiki for yourself and for others.

The best part of these guided meditations is that you can do them over and over again. If you are struggling with worry, anger, frustration, or negativity—go to your favorite meditation that helps you with those emotions. If you are working on being kinder and more grateful in your day-to-day life, use the meditations that address those issues to nurture and fine-tune those emotions.

Please—do not be a stranger.

Finally, if you found this book useful in any way, a review on Amazon is always appreciated!

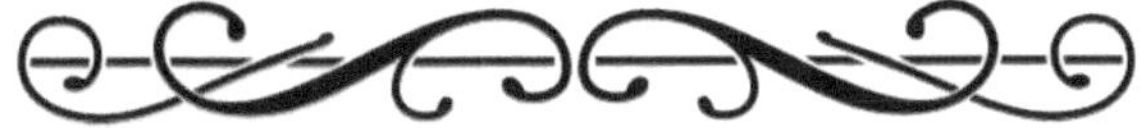